The Physicians of Myddfai

By Rhiwallon of Myddfai

Cover Design by Alex Struik

NOTICE

The medical knowledge represented in this book is over 800 years old. The publication of this book is for historical interest only, and is not to be construed as medical advice.

Medicinal plants and remedies should not be used without consulting a trained medical professional.

Medical science has made considerable progress since this book was written. Recommendations or prescriptions will have been superseded by better alternatives, or invalidated altogether.

Contents

INTRODUCTION.

1. HERE by the help of God, the supreme chief Sovereign, are shewn the most notable and principal methods of healing the human body, the persons who caused them to be written after this fashion being Rhiwallon the Physician, and his sons, even Kadwgan, Griffith, and Einion.

For they were the ablest and most eminent of the physicians of their time, and of the time of Rhys Gryg their lord, and the lord of Dinovor, the nobleman who maintained their rights and privileges, in all integrity and honour, as was meet. The reason why they thus caused a record of their skill to be committed to writing was, lest no one should be found after them so endowed with the requisite knowledge as they were.

THE HEAD.

2. The head is the first and the most important portion of man's body, which God formed, for therein are the five corporeal senses.

ORIGIN OF DISEASES IN THE HEAD.

3. Diseases originate in three places in the head; one is the pericranium, the second is the cranium, and the third is the dura mater.

PRESERVATION OF THE CRANIUM AND SCALP.

4. By an incision in the scalp, extending to the cranium,: and giving exit to the venom, is the cranium preserved. By phlebotomy and cauterization is the scalp preserved.

DURA MATER.— TREATMENT.

5. By exposing the dura mater, taking two parts of wood betony, and three parts of the violet, with salt butter, pounded together, and applying them thereto, the venom is removed from the dura mater. It will extract any inflammation and pain existing therein.

DURATION OF TREATMENT.

6. From the time the scalp is laid open to the end of nine days, shall this issue remain on the bone: that is to say, this plan should be followed in an old standing complaint of the head.

WOUND ON THE HEAD.— TREATMENT. PHYSICIAN'S FEK.

7. As to a recent blow or fresh wound on the head, the sooner it is dressed the better, lest there should be extravasated blood upon the dura mater, and that it should become concocted there. When the bone and the dura mater are exposed, take the violet and fresh butter, and pound together. If the violet cannot be gotten, take the white of eggs and linseed, pounding them together ; or fresh butter and linseed, and apply thereto till (the pain is) assuaged. Then an ointment should be prepared of herbs, butter and tallow, and applied thereto until it is cured. A pound is the physician's fee for this treatment as regards the deed of mercy simply, without victuals : or nine score (pence) with victual.

PAIN IN THE EYE. CAUTERY.

8. For pain in the eye. The actual cautery applied to the hollow of the eyebrow, and another in the nape of the neck, is beneficial for rheum of the head.

WATERY EYE.— TREATMENT.

9. For a red watery eye (ophthalmia tarsi cum epiphora) insert a seaton under the jaw, and apply the actual cautery in the nape of the neck, and this is beneficial for rheum of the head.

DISEASED KYELIUS.— REMEDY.

10. For a dry scurfy condition of the eye (lids.) Take the juice of the strawberry, a hen's fat, and May butter. Pound them well together, and keep in a horn (box.) When going

to bed, anoint (about) thine eye and eyelids well, and they will be cured.

PNEUMONIA.— TREATMENT.

11. There are three kinds of lung disease ; — simple pneumonia, white pneumonia, (bronchitis) and black pneumonia, (phthysis) which is marked by pain below the mamma?, under the armpit, and in the top of the shoulders, with (hectic) redness of the cheeks. And thus are they treated. Let (the patient) take, for three successive days, of the following herbs ; hemlock, agrimony, herb Robert, and asarabacca, then let him undergo a three day's course of aperients. When the disease is thus removed from the bronchial tubes, an emetic should be given him (daily) to the end of nine days. Afterwards let a medicine be prepared, by digesting the following herbs in wheat ale or red wine: madder, sharp dock, anise, agrimony, daisy, round birthwort, meadow sweet, yellow goat's beard, heath, water avens, woodruff, crake berry, the corn cockle, caraway, and such other herbs as will seem good to the physician. Thus is the blessed confection prepared. Take of May butter, a she-goat's suet or a doe's fat, the shepherd's needle, and as many as may be desired of such herbs as may be suitable for the purpose. A wounded lung is the physician's third difficulty, for he cannot controul it, but must wait for the will of God. By means of the herbs just mentioned, a medicine may be prepared for any one who has a pulmonary abcess (empyema.) He should let out (the matter) and support (the patient) as in the case of a wounded lung, till he is recovered. But most usually, he will have died within eleven years (al. one year.)

FEVERS.

12. There are four kinds of fevers, deriving their origin from the summer, viz. latent fever, intermittent fever, ephemeral fever, and inflammatory fever. The fifth fever is typhus, and this kind proceeds from the brain. A latent fever is relieved by an emetic, a cordial, and cauteries. Thus it originates ; from the over generating of tough humor in the stomach, from which results a distaste for food, and lassitude during summer. The mugwort, madder, meadow sweet, milfoil, hemp, red cabbage, and the tutsan, all these seven herbs enter into the composition of the medicine required. quired. Whosoever obtains them all, will not languish long from a wounded lung, or need fear for his life. Any of the following herbs may be added thereto, butcher's broom, agrimony, tutsan, dwarf elder, amphibious persicaria, centaury, round birth wort, field scabious, pepper mint, daisy, knap weed, roots of the red nettle, crake berry, St. John's wort, privet, wood betony, the roots of the yellow goat's beard, heath, water avens, woodruff, leaves of the earth nut, agrimony, wormwood, the bastard balm, small burdock, and the orpine.

INTERMITTENT FEVERS. TREATMENT.

13. For intermittent fevers. Take dandelion and fumatory, infused in water, the first thing in the morning. Then about noon take wormwood infused in water likewise, drinking it as often as ten times, the draught being rendered tepid. Let bread made with pounded wheat be also taken, or oaten cakes, goat's whey, the flesh of a young fowl, husky porridge in water, milk being abstained from, and indeed every kind of milk diet. If the ague does not then terminate, the patient must be put in a bath, when the paroxysm comes on, and an emetic given him whilst in the bath, as it will then act more powerfully.

COOLING DRINKS.

14. The three best cooling drinks are apple water, goat's whey, and spring water.

INTERMITTENT FEVERS.

15. Another treatment for an intermittent fever. Take the mugwort, dwarf elder, tutsan, amphibious persicaria, pimpernel, butcher's broom, elder bark, and the mallow, and boiling them together as well as possible in a pot, or cauldron. Then take the water and herbs, and add them to the bath. The following is a good medicine for this class of diseases : take moss, ground ivy, or elder, if obtainable, (if not obtainable, caraway,) and boil these two vegetable substances well together. Then take the mallow, fennel, pimpernel, butcher's broom, borage, and the young leaves of the earth nut, and bruise them as well as possible, putting them on the fire with the two herbs before mentioned, and boiling them well. This being done, let elder bark be taken from that portion of the tree which is in the ground,-let it be scraped and washed thoroughly, and bruised well in a mortar. Then take the liquor prepared from the fore-mentioned herbs, and mix the said bark therein assiduously between both hands, and set it to drain into a vessel to acidify, fermenting it with goat's whey, or cow's whey. Let a good cupful thereof be drank every morning as long as it lasts, a portion of raw honey, apple or wood sorrel, being taken subsequently in order to remove the taste from the mouth, after the draught. This liquor is beneficial to every man who requires to purge his body.

HEMORRHOIDS.—EXCITING CAUSE.
TREATMENT.—SURGICAL. ANOTHER

METHOD.— MEDICAL. FORBIDDEN FOOD.

16. There are two kinds of hemorrhoids, humoral hemorrhoids and inflamed hemorrhoids, the latter produced by summer heat, the former by summer moisture, when either condition prevails. It is in this manner that it comes. Four veins proceed from the liver to the anus; therefore, thus it may be cured. Secure three of these by means of a ligature, and let the fourth be left free. The cautery also should be applied to the ancles, and about the knees and hams. Thus the blood will be habitually diverted to the lower extremities, when the cauteries shall have discharged all the humor from the vein.

The second plan of treatment is as follows. Take the mallow, and boil it in wheat ale, or in spring water. Then take that which grows in the earth of the elder (bark,) bruise well in a mortar, and mix it, crude as it is, with the above mentioned decoction, and administer it quickly to the patient, so as to act upon his bowels. Let him afterwards be forbidden beef, cheese, leeks, large fish, salmon, eels, ducks, garlic, and all kinds of milk diet, except whey made with warm milk.

ABDOMINAL COMPLAINTS.- ASCITES, PERITONITIS, ABDOMINAL TUMOR, TVMPANITIS. TREATMENT OF PERITONITIS. EMETIC. EXTRACT OF STINKING HELLEBORE. INTERNAL ABDOMINAL TUMOR.— TREATMENT.

17. There are four kinds of abdominal complaints. Ascites, peritonitis, abdominal tumor, and tympanitis. Ascites cannot be cured. Tympanitis also is a disease from which there is no escape, though it is not soon fatal. Peritonitis is treated by means of an emetic, the blue confection and a medicine. These are the herbs required (for the medicine ;) the sweet gale, bay leaves, pimpernel, male speedwell, river startip, borage, moss, liverwort, the young leaves of the earth nut, and the mallow. The before-mentioned emetic should be thus prepared. Take the stinking hellebore (dug fresh) from the ground, from the root, washing it well, slicing it thin, then bruising it in a mortar, as well as can be done, the refuse being thrown away (after the juice is expressed.) The juice should then be put in a pan on the fire (and boiled) whilst there is any ebullition (till nearly solid,) keeping it by you as long as you wish, making small pills thereof when you administer it to the sick. Abdominal tumor is cured by means of cauteries, issues, a cordial, and an emetic.

ANAL WARTS.

18. Certain warts will often form about the anus. The best way to remove them, is to dig them out with cold iron, afterwards cauterizing their seat, and anointing the same with honey.

THREE KINDS OF URINARY DISORDERS. STRANGURY. HOT AIR BATH. CALCULUS—OPERATION. SUBSEQUENT TREATMENT. PREPARATORY TREATMENT. GRAVEL—TREATMENT.

19. There are three kinds of painful urinary disorders. Strangury. It is cured by means of an emetic, a cordial, cauteries, and a dry (hot air) bath. A hard vesical calculus is thus extracted by operation. Take a staff and place it in the bend of the knee ; then fix both arms within the knees, doubling them up over the staff, and securing both wrists with a fillet, over the nape of the neck, the patient (being placed on the back), his stomach up, with some support under both thighs, and the calculus cut for on the left side of the urethra. Let him be subsequently put in a water bath that same day, also the day following early, and after this he should be put in the kyffeith. Then he should be removed to his bed, and laid there on his back, his wound being cleaned, and dressed with flax and salt butter. He should be kept in the same temperature, until it be known whether he shall escape (the effects of the operation.) He should be kept without food or drink for a day and a night previous to the operation, and should have a bath. If the disease be gravel, make a medicine of the following herbs, mascerated in strong clear wheat ale, viz. water pimpernel, tutsan, meadow sweet, St. John's wort, ground ivy, agrimony, milfoil, birch, common burnet, columbine, motherwort, laurel, gromwel, betony, borage, dandelion, little field madder, amphibious persicaria, liverwort.

STERILITY.— TREATMENT.

20. A sterile woman may have a potion prepared for her by means of the following herbs, viz:—St. John's wort, yew, agrimony, amphibious persicaria, creeping cinque foil, mountain club moss, orpine and pimpernel, taking an emetic in addition.

PROFUSE MENSTRUATION.— TREATMENT.

21. A woman who is subject to profuse menstruation, should take the reddish bastard balm, small burdock, orpine, stinking goose foot, pimpernel, water avens, with the ashes of a hart's horns, that has been killed with his antlers on, boiling them, as well as possible in red wine, straining the liquor carefully, and drinking it daily, till it is finished, abstaining (the while) from stimulating food. Being restrained by the above means, the blood will be habitually diverted to the thighs and ancles.

QUINSEY.

22. The roots of the corn bell flower, will break the quinsey, being digested in cold water, drank and retained in the mouth.

EXFOLIATION OF DEAD BONE FROM THE SKULL.

23. Dandelion digested in cold water, and drank, will promote the exfoliation of the skull in aged men.

ISSUES AND SEATON'S.

24. Viper's garlic, and shepherd's needle. The juice of the roots will form an issue, that of the leaves a seaton.

ISSUES AND WORMS.

25. The roots of the mugwort boiled in wine, will form an issua also ; the leaves treated in like manner will destroy worms.

AN IMPOSTUME.

26. Comfrey root, dock root, valerian root, butter, old lard, and sulphur, pounded well together, and expressed through a cloth, are useful for an impostume.

MILK. YOUNG PORK, AND MUTTON.

27. From the time of calving up to fifteen days, cow's milk will be heating, and from thence until she is in calf, as long as she remains in profit, the milk will be heating. The flesh of a sow, under a year, and sheep flesh are watery, and for the man whose flesh is flabby in consequence of disease, such meat is not proper.

WHOLESOME MEATS.— VENISON AND PORK, PARTRDIGE AND THE HEN, FLATFISH, BASS, AND TROUT.

28. The most wholesome wild beast's flesh is venison. The most wholesome domestic animal's flesh is pork. The most wholesome wild fowl's flesh is partridge. The most wholesome domestic bird's flesh is that of the hen. The

most wholesome sea fish is the flatfish. The most wholesome fresh water fish is the bass and the trout.

ECZEMA OR HUMID TETTER.

29. For a humid tetter : honey of ivy, fox marrow, and white rosin.

TOOTHACHE.— TREATMENT.

30. For the toothache. Take the inner bark of the ivy, and the leaves of the honeysuckle, bruising them well together in a mortar, expressing them through a linen cloth into both nostrils, the patient lying on his back, and it will relieve him.

DEAFNESS. DROPS. CAUTERY.

31 . For deafness. Take a ram's urine, and eel's bile, and the juice of ash, expressing the same into the ear, and about the tooth. The actual cautery should also be applied behind the ear and angle of the jaw, a nut being inserted therein. This is a good plan.

A VIPER'S BITE. STRANGE PROPOSAL FOR EXTRACTING THE VENOM BY MEANS OF FOWLS.

32. For the bite of a viper. If the patient be a male, let a living cock be procured, and let the anal extremity be applied to the wound, and so held. This is a good plan. If the patient be a woman, let a living hen be procured and applied in the same way. This will extract the venom.

CRUSTED SCALL, OR IMPETIGO CAPITIS.

33. For a crusted scall. Take goat's dung, barley meal and red wine, boil together into a poultice, and apply to the part. This is the remedy, when the sore is not opened (by the forcible removal of the crust.)

HEADACHE, AND PAIN OF JOINTS. TREATMENT BY COUNTER IRRITATION.

34. For headache or pain in the joints. Take cakes of pounded wheat, and grind into fine meal. Then take wood sorrel, dandelion, betony, and red wine, bruising them together in a mortar well, then mixing them throughly together on the fire, adding ox tallow and salt thereto freely. Let this plaster, spread on thick cloth, be then applied to the shaven scalp. This will induce the breaking forth of boils, thereby extracting the venom, and relieving the patient.

BITE OF A SPIDER. REMEDY.

35. The bite of the spider, will not be found venomous, save from the feast of the nativity of the Virgin Mary, to that of her purification, and then by applying the yellow bed straw thereto bruised, the venom will be extracted therefrom.

WORMS. TREATMENT. FASTING.

36. For worms. Take elder bark, wallnut bark, white thorn bark, bitter sweet, and boil them together in water. Let a

cupful be drank thereof daily fasting, and let the patient abstain from food till it is almost evening. This should be repeated nine times.

A PUNCTURKD WOUND.

37. For a punctured wound. Take the dung1 of a bull, apply thereto, and it will be healed.

CARBUNCLE. SEVERAL PLANS OF TREATMENT.

38. For a carbuncle. Take St. John's wort, and apply it thereto, when first observed. Another plan is to take the flower of the knap weed or the leaves, pounding with the yolk of an egg and fine salt, then applying thereto, and this will disperse it. Another is to take the self heal, bruising it with rancid lard, and applying it thereto. Another is to take the roots of the purple dead nettle, the roots of the mugwort, and the speedwell, boiling well together in goat's milk whey, adding butter to the scum thereof, and drinking it day and night.

TREATMENT WHEN A SLOUGH IS REMOVED AFTER CARBUNCLE AND CAUTERY.

39. The treatment of a carbuncle, when the slough has been removed, or a burn (cauterization) in like circumstance. Take the wild chamomile, bake it well and powder, anointing the wound regularly, and sprinkling the powdered herbs upon it. This will produce a good and fair cicatrix. We judge that every kind of wound is benefited by milk whey,

27

ACTIVE HEMORRHAGE.

40. To restrain an active hemorrhage. Take meadowsweet, digest in cold water, and drink thereof, and this will stop it by the help of God.

HOARSENESS.

41. For hoarseness. Take the water avens, and St. John's wort, boil in pure milk, mixing butter therewith when boiling. Boil a portion thereof briskly every morning and drink.

TOOTHACHE. SEVERAL REMEDIES.

42. For the toothache. Take betony and lay it under the head, in an unbleached linen cloth, and it will cure it. Another method is to take self heal, put it in a dock leaf under the tooth, or on a hot stone, and place it hot in a cloth under the painful tooth. Another is to take the round birthwort, bruise it well, and apply it to the patient's tooth for a night. Another is to take the thorn apple and apply it well.

IMFLAMMATION OF THE MAMMA.

43. For inflammation of the mamma. Take the round birthwort and lard, apply them thereto, and they will cure it.

WORMS. REMEDY.

44. For intestinal worms. Take wine and natron, mix together and drink every morning fasting.

BITE OF A VIPER.— REMEDY. OPPROBRIUM MEDICI.

45. For the bite of a viper. Take the round birthwort, knapweed, and field scabious ; mix with water and drink. The Physician's three master difficulties are, a wounded lung, a wounded mammary gland, and a wounded knee joint.

RING WORM.

46. For the ring worm, (favus.) Take white rosin, warm it, and when soft apply it to the part. This will cure it.

SEVEN THINGS INJURIOUS TO THE EYES.

47. There are seven things hostile to the eye : weeping, watching, feasting, drunkenness, impurity, a dry film, and smoke.

THREE BONES WHICH WILL NOT UNITE WHEN FRACTURED.

48. There are three bones in a man's body, which when fractured, will never unite again, and neither of them exists when a man is born, vix, a tooth, the knee pan, and the fontenelle (or os frontis.)

TO INDUCE SLEEP.

49. Poppy heads bruised in wine, will induce a man to sleep soundly.

IMPOTENCY.

60. For impotency. Take some birch, digest in water, and drink.

INTERMITTENT FEVER. TREATMENT.

51. For intermittent fever. Take the mugwort, the purple dead nettle, and the round birthwort, as much as you like of each, bruising them well in stale goat's milk whey, and boiling afterwards. Let the patient drink some thereof every morning, and it will cure him.

TOOTHACHE. A STRANGE REMEDY, AND STRANGER PATHOLOGY.

52. For the toothache. Take a candle of sheep's suet, (some eringo seed being mixed therewith,) and burn it as near the tooth as possible, some cold water being held under the candle. The worms (destroying the tooth) will drop into the water, in order to escape from the heat of the candle.

A TUMOR OF THE ABDOMEN.— POULTICE. TUMOR OF THE ABDOMEN AGAIN.

53. For a tumor of the abdomen. Take sheep's suet, oatmeal, foxglove, and pimpernel, making a poultice of them, and apply it thereto. If it contains matter this will bring it to a head.

For a tumor of the abdomen again. Take goat's milk whey, being fresh, mix ramsons therewith, and drink of it for three days, and the swelling will disappear.

FALLING FITS. TREATMENT, ROUGH, BUT READY.

54. For falling fits. Burn a goat's horn, directing the smoke upon the patient, and in consequence of the smell he will forthwith arise. Before he has risen from the ground, apply dog's gall upon his head, and that disease will not attack him any more.

INTERMITTENTS OR AGUES. A STRANGE MODE OF PROGNOSTIC.

55. For all sorts of agues, write in three apples, on three separate days. 1n the first apple [+] o nagla pater. 1n the second apple [+] o nagla filius. 1n the third apple [+] nagla spiritm sanctas. And on the third day he will recover. If you would know how it will happen to a man who sickens, whether he will live or die of his disease, take the herb called violet, bruise it, and bind a portion to both legs, and if the patient will live, he will sleep, and if he cannot sleep, he will die.

TO PREVENT INTOXICATION. TO PREVENT WEARINESS.

56. If you would not be drunk, drink in the morning as much as will fill an egg-shell of the juice of the hemp agrimony.

If you would not be weary on a journey, drink in the morning an egg-shell full of the juice of mugwort and garlic, and you will neither be hurt nor tired, whatever distance you may walk that day.

DRUNKENNESS. TO REMOVE.

57. If you would remove a man's drunkenness, let him eat bruised saffron with spring water.

HOW TO BE MERRY.

58. If you would be at all times merry, eat saffron in meat or drink, and you will never be sad : but beware of eating over much, lest you should die of excessive joy.

TO CURE ENVY.

59. If you would never be in an envious mood, drink as much as would fill an egg shell of the juice of the herb called wild clary, and you will not after fall into an evil temper. If you would be always in good health, drink a spoonful of the juice of the herb mallows, and you will always be so.

TO PRESERVE CHASTITY.

60. If you would always bo chaste, eat daily some of the. herb called hart's tongue, and you will never assent to the suggestions of impurity.

PROLAPSUS UTERI. TREATMENT.

61. For prolapsus of the womb (that is an extrusion thereof.) The best remedy is to take wheaten flour, and knead it with the yolks of nine eggsi and honey, working into it the breast fur of two hares ; then bake it under ashes, and (making a potion thereof) drink it till the organ returns.

TOOTHACHE. TO PREVENT.

62. If you would always be free from toothache, whenever you wash, rub the inside of your ears with your fingers.

SMALL TUMOR. A FOWL APPLICATION.

63. For a small tumor. Take a cock or hen, (as the patient may be a man or a woman,) and apply the rump feathered, to the part, till the bird dies. This will extract the venom.

WARTS. TO REMOVE.

64. Whosoever would remove warts, let him apply daisy bruised in dog's urine thereto, and they will all disappear.

FLEAS. TO DESTROY.

65. Whosoever would destroy fleas, let him steep wormwood in the sea for an hour, and afterwards dry it in the sun. When sufficiently dry, any fleas coming in contact therewith will die.

FLIES. TO DESTROY.

66. To destroy flies, let the mugwort be put in the place where they frequent, and such of them as shall come in contact with the herb will die.

BITE OF A VIPER.

67. For the bite of a snake. Let the juice of the elder be drank, and it will disperse all the poison.

LOSS OF REASON OR SPEECH.

68. Whosoever shall have lost his reason or his speech, let him drink of the juice of the primrose, within two months afterwards, and he will indeed recover.

STRANGE DIAGNOSTIC OF PREGNANCY.

69. Whosoever would know whether a woman be enceinte with a boy or girl, let him observe her sitting and standing, and if she moves the right foot first it signifies a son, but if the left, a daughter.

STRANGE DIAGNOSTIC OF VIRGINITY.

70. If you would distinguish between a wife and a virgin, scrape some jet into water, and give it her to drink. If she be a wife, she will without fail pass water, but if a virgin she will not have a more urgent call than usual.

TO SILENCE A COCK.

71. If you should wish that a cock should not crow, anoint his crest with oil, and he will be mute.

OPACITY OF THE EYE.

72. For an opacity of the eye. Let some ground ivy juice be put therein, and the opacity will be removed, the eye becoming spotless and clear.

A WEEPING CHILD.

73. Let the two lower extremities of the babe, much given to weeping, be anointed with hart's marrow, and he will weep the less.

TO REMOVE A SMALL TUMOR

74. Should a man have a small tumor in a dangerous part of his body, and you should wish to remove it, your object can thus be accomplished. Take the leaves of the foxglove, and press them well on any part (of the tumor,) and it will remove it an inch and a half from the herb.

HYGEIAN OF THE YEAR.

JANUARY.

75. Month of January. Do not bleed. Drink three cupfuls of wine, fasting. Take a potion. Let your diet be goat's flesh and wholesome vegetables.

FEBRUARY.

76. Month of February. Bleed from the thumb of the left hand. Obtain a confection and a potion, which will render your eyes healthy.

MARCH.

77. Month of March. Use enemata, the roots of vegetables, and the bath. Do not bleed frequently. Do not take an emetic, as it generates cold within. Drink sweet wine, fasting.

APRIL.

78. Month of April. Bleed. Take a gentle emetic, eat fresh meat, use warm drink. Eat two mouthfuls of hart's tongue twice a day. Avoid the roots of vegetables, as they will occasion an obstruction. Drink hemp agrimony.

MAY.

79. Month of May. Do not eat sheep's head or trotters, use warm drink. Eat twice daily of hart's tongue, fasting. Take a gentle emetic. Use cold whey. Drink of the juice of fennel and wormwood.

JUNE.

80. Month of June. Take a cupful of cold water, fasting daily. Do not drink ale or mead. Drink milk warm, and eat lettuce.

JULY.

81. Month of July. Do not bleed. Take an emetic. Make use of flowers and wholesome vegetables. Avoid impurity.

AUGUST.

82. Month of August. Make use of soups and vegetables. Drink neither ale nor mead. Take white pepper in gruel.

SEPTEMBER.

83. Month of September. Take three draughts of milk the first thing in the morning daily. You may after this take what you wish, for vegetables and fruit are then ripe, and bread apt to be mouldy.

OCTOBER.

84. Month of October. Make use of new wine. Eat minnows. Take an emetic. Let your diet consist of fresh meat and vegetables of a wholesome nature.

NOVEMBER.

85. Month of November. Do not take butter, as at this time (of the year,) the blood of all men has a tendency to coagulation, which is dangerous. At this time also the heads

of beasts and all vegetables are to be avoided, being unwholesome.

DECEMBER.

86. Month of December. Do not drink soup or eat the red cabbage in the soup, nor trotters (sheep's,) and reduce your blood.

A GOOD DAY TO BLEED.

87. Whoever is bled on the 17th of March, will not be liable to intermittents or cough in that year.

SAME.

88. Whosoever is bled on the 3rd day of April, will not suffer from disease, from the head to the coccyx, in that same year, unless he is subjected to (undue) abstinence.

SAME.

89. The llth day of the same month is also a good time to be bled, so also is the 4th and 5th day of May.

SAME.

90. Whosoever is bled on the 17th day of September, will not be attacked by colic, ague, nor cough that year.

DANGEROUS DAYS TO BLEED.

91. Whosoever is bled on the third Monday in January, the first Monday in February, and the second Monday of October, will be in danger of death. There are three days in the year in which no bleeding should take place, nor any medicinal potion taken, even the last day of April, the first Monday of August, and the last Monday in September.

THINGS TO BE AVOIDED.

92. Whosoever is bled on those days, will die by the 15th or 7th day. And this is the reason. The veins will be full in those days, and if any medicinal potion is taken, it will be

dangerous. And if he eats of the flesh of a goose, he will die on the third day, or else will be an invalid in a fortnight, or else he will die in the days mentioned of sudden death.

DANGEROUS DAYS IN THE YEAR.

93. Sound teachers have discovered and written as follows, namely, that thirty t wo days in the year are dangerous. Know that whosoever is born on one of those days, will not live long, and whosoever is married on one of them, will die ere long, or will only exist in pain and poverty. And whosoever shall begin business on one of them, will not complete it satisfactorily ; and those days are : —

In JANUARY there are seven, even 1st, 2nd, éth, 5th, 10th, 15th, 17th.
In FEBRUARY there are three, — 16th, 17th, 18th.
In MARCH there are three, — 15th, 16th, 18th.
In APRIL there are two, — 3rd and 16th.
In MAY there are four,— 15th, 16th, 17th, 20th.
In JUNE there is one, — 2nd.
In JULY there are two, — 15th and 17th.
In Auoust there are two, — 18th and 20th.
In SEPTEMBER there are two, — 16th and 18th.
In OCTOBER there is one, — 6th.
In NOVEMBER there are two, — 15th and 20th.
In DECEMBER there are three, — 16th, 17th, 18th.
The eighth, at noon.
The ninth, at all times.
The tenth.
The eleventh, in the evening.
The twelfth, at all times.
The thirteenth, at all times.
The fourteenth, at all times.
The sixteenth, in the morning.
Thes eventeenth.
The eighteenth, at the third hour.
Unlucky or dangerous days. The twentieth, after dusk. The twenty third. The twenty fourth, before noon. The twenty flfth, at vesper time. The twenty sixth, at all times. The

twenly seventh. The twenty eighth, in the evening. The twenty ninth. The thirtieth.

January, 1st, 2nd, 4th, 5th, 10th, 12th, 19th.
February, 7th, 14th, 18th.
March, 15th, 16th, 18th.
April, 6th, 11th.
May, 5th, 6th, 16tb, 20th.
June, 12th. July, 15th, 20th.
August, 2nd, 12th, 19th.
September, 16th, 17th.
October, 5th.
November, 7th, 16th, 20th.
December, 6th, 8th, 15th.

Whosoever doubts these sayings, let him know that he is wiser than those who obtained this knowledge first.

SWELLING OF STOMACH.

94. For swelling or hardness of the stomach. Boil duckweed in goat's milk, and foment it therewith frequently.

SWELLING AND PAIN IN THE LOWER EXTREMITIES.

95. For swelling or pain in the lower extremities. Take the roots of tutsan and the bark thereof, boiling them in water, and when boiled pour off the supernatant liquor, and take the residuum and mix with old lard. Then spread on a cloth or a handkerchief, and apply to the swollen feet or legs, and it will be dispersed.

SWELLING AND PAIN IN THE NAPE OF THE NECK.—TREATMENT.

96. For swelling or pain in the nape of the neck. Pound the roots of celandine in a mortar, with fennel, garlic, vinegar or wine, and butter, binding the same about your neck, and it will remove the pain and disperse the swelling.

EPISTAXIS.

97. For bleeding of the nose. Boil garlic in milk and water and drink it. 1t is proved.

BURNS. A CAPITAL PLASTER. ANOTHER GOOD ONE. ANOTHER AGAIN.

98. For burns occurring in any part of the body. Take the root of the white lily, and wash clean, boiling it briskly in water. Then reduce to a pulp, and mix with oil, and a little white of eggs, spreading it on lint. Let this be applied night and morning. The more plaster you apply the better.

Another mode. Burn ivy in a clean place, and cover the burn with the ashes of the same, and it will heal it presently. Another way is to burn fern, and mix the ashes with the white of eggs ; or else oil, anointing the burn with it. and it will heal it quickly and wonderfully.

NETTLE RASH, OR ERYSEPELATOUS ERETHEMA. TREATMENT.

99. A medicine for nettle rash, (when indicating a bad constitution,) so that it may disappear in three days. Take good cheese and pound it briskly in a mortar. Mix honey with it till it is transparent. Anoint the part therewith frequently, laying a cabbage leaf thereon, and it will have disappeared in three days.

BITE OF A MAD DOG. TREATMENT.

100. For the bite of a mad dog. Pound ground ivy well in a mortar with lard, or pound leeks and vinegar, or fennel seed, and honey together, and apply thereto.

INFLAMMATION OF MAMMAE.

101. For inflammation of the mammae. Pound the roots of the tutsan with rancid lard, and apply thereto.

INSANITY.—TO CURE.

102. When a man becomes insane, take daisy, field southernwood and sage, digesting it in wine, and let the patient drink it for fifteen days.

OBSTINATE CONSTIPATION.—TO OVERCOME.

103. If the bowels become so constipated that they cannot be moved, take duckweed, boiling it briskly in a pot, then cast it into a pan, and fry with a quantity of blood and butter, eating it hot.

PALSY.- TO CURE.

104. For the palsy. Take the field southernwood, pound it in a mortar, and strain the juice to about a small cupful, and give it the patient to drink, on the dawn of God's day of Christmas.

BLEEDING OF THE NOSE.—REMEDY.

105. For bleeding of the nose. Take as much as you can hold between your three fingers of the betony, being briskly powdered with salt, and put it in your nostrils, which will stop it quickly.

ADHESION OF THE LIVER.— TREATMENT.

106. If a man's liver should adhere to his ribs, take in the morning at sun rise, (chanting thy pater noster,) some river star tip. Digest it in new ale, and give it the patient to drink (whilst in a bath,) for nine days.

COUGH.—REMEDY. ANOTHER METHOD.

107. For a cough. Bruise hemp agrimony, in a mortar, and mix the juice with boiling milk, strain and use. Another method. Boil a potful of water until it is wasted to the half. Then mix rye meal therewith, and add butter, eating it hot.

WORMS.—TO DESTROY. ANOTHER METHOD.

108. To destroy worms in the stomach or bowels. Take the juice of turnips, foment therewith, and they will come out.

Another method is to take a handful of the bark of the peach tree, growing in dry ground, drinking it fasting with goat's milk, and they will all come out.

CONSTIPATION.— TO OVERCOME.— SUPPOSITORY.

109. To overcome constipation. Take salt and second milk, equal parts of each, put on the fire in an evaporating dish, leaving it there until it is reduced into a soft waxlike mass. Then make cakes (suppositories) of the same, and pass them into the patient's rectum.

BITE OP A SNAKE.— ANTIDOTES FOR. ANOTHER WAY.

110. For the bite of a snake. Drink the juice of the greater plantain, with oil and salt. The juice of the mugwort also', when bruised and strained will neutralize poison. Another way is to take the brains of a red cock and rue; mix with sweet milk, curdled milk or wine, and drink. Take also of the flesh of the breast whilst warm, (the cock being alive,) and apply to the wound. It will extract the venom.

WORMS.— A CATAPLASM.— A REMEDY. ANOTHER.

111. For worms. Take the milk of a cow, that has a bull calf sucking her, with barley meal and honey. Boil it in a pan after the manner of porridge, and apply hot to the stomach.

Another method is to make bread of barley and the kernels of nuts, (shelled,) eating it.

Another plan is to bruise fresh rue and mugwort in a mortar, and drink the juice thereof.

DIFFICULT PARTURITION.— TO HELP.

112. If a woman be unable to give birth to her child, let the mugwort be bound to her left thigh. Let it be instantly removed when she has been delivered, lest there should be hemorrhage.

SWELLING AND PAIN OP LEGS.— AN APPLICATION FOR.

113. For swelling and pain in the thighs. Bruise rue, honey, and salt, apply thereto, and it will disperse the swelling.

PAIN IN THE KIDNEYS.— A REMEDY.

114. For pain in the kidneys. Take the centaury, infused in cold water, and give it to the patient to drink.

EXTREME THIRST,— TO HELP.

115. For extreme thirst. Drink the centaury infused in hot water. This will quench thirst, and clear the breast and stomach.

SMALL POX.— AN APPLICATION.

116. For the small pox. Take the ashes of heath, balm or smallage, and the ashes of hartshorn, with honey, and anoint therewith.

A SURFEIT.— TO RELIEVE.

117. For a surfeit. Take turnip, boil in goafs milk, and let the patient drink thereof, and he will be relieved.

A BURN OR SCALD.— A FOMENTATION FOR.

118. For a burn or scald. Put the leaves of the lily, in boiling milk, and apply to the part till it is well.

RETENTION OF URINE.— A STRANGE REMEDY.

119. For retention of urine. Take the brains of a hare, and mix the same with wine. Let the patient smell it for an hour and then drink it.

BITE OP A V[PER.— REMEDY.

120. For the bite of an adder. Mix the juice of the fennel, of radish, rue or wormwood, with oil, let the patient drink the same, or eat it.

VOMITING OF BLOOD.— REMEDIES.

121. For vomiting of blood. Boil the milfoil with wine or milk, and drink, as this will stop it. Or boil the betonica in goat's milk, or wine, and this will restrain it.

CONSTIPATION.— REMEDY FOR.

122. For constipation. Boil roots of the small thistles, growing in woods, and give the water to the patient to drink

FATNESS.— TO REDUCE.

123. Whosoever is over fat, let him drink of the juice of the fennel, and it will reduce him.

IRRITABILITY OF MIND.— TO CALM.

124. If a man be irritable of mind, let him drink of the juice of the apinm, (celery) frequently, as it will relieve him of his irritability, and produce joy.

REPTILES IN THE STOMACH.— TO EXPEL THEM.

125. If a snake should enter a person's mouth, or there should be any other living reptiles in him, let him take wild camomile, (in powder,) in wine, till it is thickned, and drink the same, as it will relieve him of them.

WORMS IN MAN OR BEAST.— TO KILL. ANOTHER PLAN.

126. If worms be generated in man or beast, apply to (his stomach,) the roots of the taragon, and the worm will die forthwith.

Another way is to mix the leaves of the dittany with strong wine, and let the patient drink it fasting.

INTESTINAL WORMS.— REMEDY. ANOTHER.

127. For intestinal worms. Let the patient drink a cupful of the juice of the plantain, and apply the same herb to the navel.

Another way is to take milfoil in wine, once whilst fasting, and they will bo expelled that day.

AGUE.— A REMEDY WITH A PATER NOSTER. ANOTHER REMEDY.

128. For the ague. Drink the juice of rue in wine, swallow three grains of coriander, drink celery (apium) in water, (sweetened,) and collect plantain whilst saying your pater

noster, and drink it infused in wine and pepper. Take the juice of the mugwort bruised, the juice of the wormwood, and tepid oil. Then anoint your whole body on one side three days successively, and it will cure the aguo for you cheaply.

AN OBSTINATE AGUE.— TREATMENT.

129. But if a man has indeed an obstinate ague, cause him to go into a bath, and let him avoid touching the water with his arms. Let him also take ground ivy, boiling it briskly, and apply hot to his head. He must also be bled in his arm, and he will be cured by the help of God.

VOMITING AND SIGHING.— A REMEDY.

130. For vomiting and sighing. Mix a handful and a half of betony in warm water, and drink it.

To cure vomiting, take betonica, and boil in honey, pounding in a mortar, and form into four balls, and administer to him one daily as a drink, in a warm potion.

POISON,— ANTI DOTE.

131. If a man has taken poison let him take of the juice of the dittany, and wine.

BLEEDING PROM THE NOSE.— REMEDY. ANOTHER.

132. To stop bleeding from the nose, take the tops of three nettles, pounding them together. Put this cataplasm on the nape of your neck, and if possible in your nostrils. Another

method is to pound the milfoil with vinegar in a mortar. Plug the nostrils therewith, and it will stay the bleeding.

VOMITING.— STRANGE TREATMENT.

133. For vomiting. Drink milfoil digested in warm wine, till a cure is obtained.

Another plan is to immerse the scrotum in vinegar.

DEAFNESS AFTER FEVER.

134. For deafness succeeding a fever; take a cow's gall, a woman's milk, and honey, putting it in your ears warm. This is a cure that will not fail.

MANIFOLD VIRTUES OF THE LEEK.

135. The following are the virtues of the leek. It is good to drink the juice against vomiting of blood. 1t is good for women who desire children to eat leeks. 1t is good to take leeks and wine for the bite of an adder, or other (venomous) beast. 1t is good to apply a plaster of leeks and wine to ulcers. The juice of leeks and woman's milk is a good remedy for a chronic whooping cough, or pneumonia. The juice of leeks, goat's gall, and honey, mixed in three equal parts, are useful for deafness. 1t should be put warm in the ears and nostrils. It is good for headache. Leeks are good to promote the union of bones, and maturing of boils. If leeks and salt are applied to ulcers, it will heal them rapidly. If leeks are eaten raw, they will occasion intoxication. They will strengthen men who have suffered from hemorrhage. They will relieve flatulency of the stomach. They are oppressive to the stomach, whether boiled or raw, as they will destroy the nervous energy thereof, and their fumes

rising to the head, injure the sight. They produce terrific dreams. Unless the lettuce or the poppy, or the like are eaten first to temperate them, such is their tendency. They kill the worms that are generated in the stomach or bowels.

VOMITING.— TO STAY.

136. Those that cannot retain food or drink, but vomit it, the milfoil digested in warm wine, should be given them to drink.

ANTIDOTE TO POISON.

137. As an antidote for poison, mix two nuts, three dry figs, and a handful of rue, and thirty grains of salt, giving it to the patient, fasting.

PROUD FLESH.— APPLICATION.

138. The following is useful when proud flesh forms in a wound, namely, white alum, reduced to powder, the same powder being applied thereon.

Another for the same purpose. Take a toad that can scarcely creep, beat it with a rod, till irritated, it smells, and dies. Then put it in an earthen pot, closing the same so that no smoke can come out, or air enter in. Then burn it till it is reduced to ashes, and apply the same to the part.

ANOTHER WAY.

Another plan is to take a mole, (al. raven,) and burn it in the same way, applying the ashes upon the part.

ANOTHER.

In like manner, make ashes of human flesh, taken if possible from a corresponding part of the body to that in which the disease is situated.

PROUD FLESH.— ANOTHER APPLICATION.

In like manner you may take the ashes of the ermine, burnt in the way above mentioned, and apply thereto.

ANOTHER.

Another plan is to take as many as you please of the cloves of garlick, burning them on a clean floor ; when they are incinerated, quench (the fire) with drops of honey, make a powder thereof, and apply. Bind it over with a plaster, and in three days afterwards let it be washed. Boil rye meal and a sow's blood together, applying it thereon when it is worked; over that a plaster of boiling honey, and a third part of salt should be applied. Do this daily.

ANOTHER.

Another plan is to take the jaw of a horse, with all the teeth remaining therein. Burn a cupful thereof (in powder,) and mix with pepper and lard : anoint the part with this, tempering with sage. Continue to apply this plaster daily, for a fortnight.

ANOTHER.

Another is to take honey, the yolk of an egg, good milk, and fine confectioner's meal, mix together and apply to the part twice daily. This is proved.

VIRTUES OF MUSTARD.

139. Mustard. It is useful to expel cold humors. It is good with vinegar for the bite of an adder or toad. It is good for the toothache. It will purify the brain. It will restrain profuse menstruation. It will provoke the appetite, and strengthen digestion. It is good for colic, loss of hair, noise in the ears, and dimness of sight, cutaneous eruptions, palsy, and many other things.

URINAL PATHOLOGY.— FOUR URINARY ELEMENTS.

140. From the condition of a man's urine, may be distinguished his defects, dangers, fevers (plagues,) and diseases, whether he be present or absent. However, we should first show what is the composition of the urine. It contains four radical elements.

FIRST. The humor of the blood which circulates in the reproductive organs.
The following are the elementary rules of urinoscopy. If the urine exhibits a yellow colour of a faint golden hue, or if it has the hue of refined gold ; it indicates that food and drink are perfectly digested in the stomach.

If of a fiery red, like the sunset in the west — if red like oriental saffron — if a fiery red like a vanishing flame — if red like a portion of consuming tire ; these four colours indicate that the food and drink have left the stomach iu order that their digestion may be completed.

If urine is deep coloured like human liver, or the hue of (blushing) cheeks, like racked red wine, or greenish like the mane of oxen ; these three colours concur in indicating that food and drink are properly digested in the stomach.

If water has a leaden hue, or an intensely black colour like black ink, or a dead black, like black horn ; these three colours indicate the death of a man.

If it has the colour of clear spring water, if an opaline colour like transparent horn, or the colour of plain milk, or the hue of camel hair ; these four colours indicate the nondigcstion of the food in the stomach.

If it has a greenish blue colour, this indicates that less food and drink should be allowed the patient.

If the colour of ill bled meat, it indicates that the digestion of food has commenced in the stomach.

If a greenish hue like an unripe apple, — if the hue of a ripe apple ; these two colours indicate that the food and drink are half digested in the stomach. And thus it terminates."

SECONDLY. That of the abdominal viscera for the performance of the functions thereof.

THIRDLY. That of the vessels which receive the various fluids of the cholera and fleuma (bile and phlegm).

FOURTHLY. That of the kidneys, supplying those fluids which pass to the bladder. From hence can be discerned all the signs of disease, the fluidity and colour of the urine indicating the evil and good signs.

URINAL DIAGNOSIS.

141. Should urine abound in water, or resemble red, black, or green wine, or oil, or blood, or the urine of beasts, and a skilful person consider the essential causes thereof, attentively studying the same, he will understand which of these humors chiefly predominate, whether the fleuma, the cholera, the sanguis, or the melancholia. It is necessary that the urine be collected in a glass vessel, and left to settle till the second hour, when, by the light of the sun, the physician should judge the indications thereof.

SIGNS IN ORDER.—

BLACK URINE.

i. If the urine be black, it will be necessary to renovate that patient's constitution by the most skilful means possible, frequently employing the bath and oil. Then the urine should be again examined, and if it should seem saffron-like and turbid, know that there is a painful disease in the person, produced by heat and dryness.

SINOPLE.

ii. If the patient be attenuated and evidently declining in strength, his veins prominent, or red (transparent,) and the urine similar in colour to sinople, it proceeds frum the sanguis. By bleeding the patient in the left arm, he will be restored with little trouble.

THICK, OILY, OPAQUE AND SANGUINOLENT.

iii. If the urine should be thick, oily, deep red, not transparent in the rays of the sun, and sanguinolent, it indicates languishment and weakness of body, from excess of fever.

CURDLED.

iv. If the urine be curdled, it indicates a long continued fever.

RED AND CHANGEABLE.

v. If the urine be red, or brimstone-like, and seeming to change its appearance frequently, it indicates a dangerous fever.

CLOUDY AND GREENISH.— A CLOUD ON THE SURFACE.

vi. If the urine bo cloudy and greenish at the commencement of a fever, or in two days afterwards, when secreted it seems thicker and thicker, the patient is sure to die. If these signs increase in number, though the urine does not thicken, it indicates a tedious fever.

If there be a sky appearance on the surface of the urine, it indicates a future fever.

FOUL URINE.

vii. If the urine seem foul in fever, it indicates heat and blindness, pain of head and shoulders, with deafness. If the patient is not relieved in seven days, he will die.

OILY.

viii. If the urine seems like oil during the heat of a fever, it indicates death, delirium or erysipelas. If it is not • juickly removed, it indicates a softening of the brain.

FIERY, AND PASSED WITH PAIN.

ix. If it assumes a fiery hue, and is passed with pain, this indicates that the patient's food and drink are not properly digested. It is accordingly expedient in such a case for the patient to restrict himself to spoon diet.

BLACK OR RED, WITH SEDIMENT.

x. If it be black or red, and there be sediment in the bottom, with retention, pain in the kidneys, and pain in micturition, the patient is in danger. If the urine be passed frequently, and in small quantities, then it indicates a stone in the bladder.

BLUISH WHITE, &c.

xi. If the urine be bluish white, during the heat of a fever, or reddish brown or red, accompanied with bleeding at the nose, it is attended with great danger.

WHITE.

xii. In persons with a diseased liver, when thin urine becomes white, it indicates future agony, but if it disappears suddenly, it indicates a boil.

BILIOUS.

xiii. If in the heat of a fever it has the colour of bile, being thick, with a whitish cloud and whitish granules floating thereon, it indicates a long continued languishing.

xiv. If more is passed than is proper, during the heat of a fever, and the colour is not good, though passed freely, it indicates danger at hand. If the urine is not natural, when passed, and it subsequently assumes a healthy colour, it indicates that the patient will pine away from future torment.

xv. If a man in the heat of a fever passes his urine sufficiently natural, but with white gravel therein, the fever not decreasing, it indicates danger.

xvi. If it abounds in water, the fever will increase, but he will be in no danger.

xvii. If the urine be dark, during the heat of a fever, the turbidness not subsiding, his illness will resolve itself into an ague in four, or perhaps three days.

xviii. If it be red, with much sediment, it will indicate a fever.

xix. If it has the colour of water, the fever will increase, but there will be no danger.

xx. Urine during the heat of a fever, if it be viscid and filthy, abounding with a gravelly sediment, with a cloudiness on the surface, indicates a tedious illness.

xxi. The urine of fever having sandy sediment, being sanguinolent in colour within, indicates disease of the kidneys.

xxii. If the urine should be frothy, like bubbles on water, let him not be surprised at the occurrence of any disease, as it indicates a fever at hand.

xxiii. If the urine be white in the morning, and afterwards red, it is well. 1t only signifies the proper flux of the body.

xxiv. If it be red first, and afterwards black, or if the urine has a mixture of those two colours, it indicates death.

xxv. If it be greasy on the surface, bubbles ascending therein, it is a bad sign.

xxvi. If it be greasy on the surface, and white sediment in the bottom of the vessel, it indicates pain in the viscera or joints.

xxvii. If the urine be blue, it indicates a disease of the viscera.

xxviii. An ill looking red urine, containing a gravelly sediment, and having a cloudiness on the surface, is a bad sign.

xxix. If it be very white, it is unfavourable. If it is dark in the morning, so much the worse.

xxx. If it be greasy, and preceded by great pain, it is indicative of death. If it be transparent, with a cloudiness thereon, the death of that patient will be nigh at hand. If it be light coloured in the morning, and lighter after dinner, it will be all the better. If it be red with a sediment, it indicates no danger. A dark hepatic urine indicates danger.

A pale splenetic urine is dangerous. A red urine from dyspepsia is dangerous. A clear urine indicates a healthy condition. And thus it ends.

BLEEDING.

142. In bleeding, the blood should be permitted to flow till the colour changes, and the stream of blood from black should flow till it is red. If thick, let it flow till it becomes more fluid. If it is watery, let it flow till it becomes thicker.

HEALTH.

143. To secure constant health, drink daily, the first thing, a spoonful of the juice of the mallows.

BIRDS AND FLIES.

144. To drive away birds or flies, put the mugwort in the places where they frequent, and they will disperse.

SPECK IN THE EYE.

145. For a speck in the eye, put therein the juice of the ground ivy.

INTOXICATION.

146. In order to be delivered from intoxication, drink saffron digested in spring water.

A TUMOR.

147. For a tumor. Apply a cock or a hen thereto till the animal dies.

FALLING SICKNESS.

148. For falling sickness. Let a dog be killed, and, unknown to the patient, put some of the gall in his mouth. It will never attack him again.

PROGNOSIS OF DEATH.

149. In order to form a prognosis of the fate of a sick person, bruise the violet, apply to the eyebrows, and if he sleeps, he will live, but if not, he will die.

CHASTITY.

150. If you would preserve yourself from unchaste desires, eat rue in the morning.

URINARY CALCULI.— TO DISSOLVE.

151. To destroy urinary calculi. Take saxifrage, which grows in stony places, (it has obtained its name from its virtues in this respect,) temper with wine and pepper, drinking it warm. This will break the stone, and promote the passing of water. It will also promote menstruation, and cure diseases of the kidneys and uterus.

AGAIN.

Another way (of dissolving the stone) is to take the saxifrage and the seed of the gromwell, digesting them in boiling water. Let the patient drink this for six days, and he will be cured without fail.

AGAIN.— EXPERIMENT.

Another mode is to take the blood and skin of a hare, burning them to ashes. Then mix a quantity of this powder in warm water, and let the patient drink a spoonful of the mixture, fasting, and it will disintegerate the stone, causing it to be expelled. If you would wish to prove this, put a spoonful of the same powder in water, and deposit any calculus you please therein, and it will instantly slacken it.

THREE THICK INCURABLE ORGANS.

152. There are three thick incurable organs ; the liver, kidney, and heart. The reason why they are so called is that when disease has aflected either of them, no relief can be given, but a painful death.

THREE THIN INCURABLE ORGANS.

153. There are three thin incurable organs; the pia mater, small intestines, and bladder. They are incurable for the same cause as the others.

THREE COMPLAINTS WHICH OCCASION CONFINEMENT.

154. There are three complaints which occasion long confinement. Disease of the knee joint, of the substance of

a rib, and of a lung. For when matter has formed in either, a surgeon does not know when he may be cured till he sees him well.

HEMORRHOIDS.

155. For hemorrhoids. Apply the calcareous droppings of peacocks (pounded) with fern roots, and it will cure it.

HYDROPHOBIA.

156. The bite of a mad dog. It is a good thing to eat the root of radish.

BARRENNESS CURED.

157. To render a woman fruitful, let her frequently eat lettuce, hot tallow, and pepper.

GREATEST REMEDY.

158. What is the greatest remedy (or effort of surgical skill ?) To remove a bone from the brain (to trephine) with safety.

LEAST REMEDY.

159. What is the simplest remedy? To scratch one's hand until it is irritated, and then to spit upon it forthwith.

PAIN.

160. An antidote for pain: seek the dittany, which may be obtained from cunning men; it is the best in all complaints.

A TUMOR.— REMEDY.

161. For a tumor. Take the daisy and plantain (in powder,) mixing the same with drink, till it is thickened. Take also dust scraped from blue stone (sulphate of copper,) and administer to him in drink. It will cure him, if it is given him ere he sleeps.

SWELLING AFTER INJURY.— REMEDY.

162. For a swelling, the result of an injury. Take the juice of the yellow bed straw, the juice of the plantain, rye meal, honey and the white of eggs. Make into a plaster, and apply thereto.

BOILS.

163. For boils. Take the juice of the morella (mushroom,) plantain, barley meal, and the white of an egg.

STRANGURY.

164. For strangury. Take the dead red nettle, and parsley. Make a plaster thereof, and apply to the stomach below the navel.

WARTS.

165. To remove warts. Take the inner bark of the willow, make into a plaster with vinegar, and apply it.

HEARTACHE.

166. For the heartache. Take the bark of the keginderw, the bark of the stinking goose foot, the plantain, and the shepherd's purse, boiling them in ditch (stagnant) water. till it is wasted to a third. Take this water and make it into a gruel, with wheaten flour.

Another way is to take caraway water and goat's milk in equal parts, mixing plantain juice therewith, and boiling river granite therein. Let this be given the patient nine days, unmixed with any other drink.

DYSPEPSIA.

167. For pain in the chest (dyspepsia.) Take a large quantity of black thorn berries, bruise briskly in a mortar, mixing very new ale therewith. Put this mixture in a new earthen pot, over its edges in the earth, for nine days and nights, giving it the patient to drink the first thing in the morning, and the last thing at night.

TO MAKE VINEGAR.

168. To make vinegar. Take clean barley, and put in wine over night till the eve of next day.

TO PROMOTE THE UNION OF BONE.

169. To promote the union of bone. Take comfrey, and bruise with wine, pepper and honey, drinking it daily for nine days, and they will unite compactly.

EYE SALVE.

170. To make an eye salve. Take the juice * * * and the juice of fennel root, celandine, lesser celandine, sow's lard, honey, a little vinegar, an eel's1 blood, and a cock's gall, letting them stand in a brass vessel till an efflorescence takes place. This has restored sight to those who had quite lost it.

DIGNITY OF MEDICINE.

171. Let all men know that it will be vain to seek anything except by effort. There can be no effort without health ; there can be no health without temperance in a man's nature, and temperance cannot exist in a man's nature without moderate heat in his extremities. God has decreed a supervision of the manner in which we should conserve the health, and has revealed it to his own servants, the philosophers and chosen prophets, who are full of the Holy Spirit, and whom God ordained to this profession.

172. The Latins, the men of Persia and the Greeks (say,) what we choose we love, what we seek we think of. Therefore let all men know that God has given the men of Greece a special gift, to discern every art, and the nature of all things, to a greater extent than other nations, with a view to the preservation of human health.

173. The philosophers and wise men foreknew that man was formed of four elements, each being antagonistic to the

others, and each consequently requiring continual aliment, which if it do not obtain, it will succumb. If a man partakes of too much or too little food or drink, the body will rbecome weak, fall into disease, and be open to injurious consequences. If he partakes temperately of food and drink, the body will acquire strength, and the health will also be preserved.

MODERATION.

174. The philosophers have said whosoever shall eat or drink more or less than he should, or shall sleep more or less, or shall labour more or less from idleness or from hardship, (being obliged to over exert himself :) or who, used to being bled, refrains from doing so, without doubt he will not escape sickness. Of these things we shall treat presently, and of what is most suitable for our use.

SAYINGS OF THE WISE AS TO FOOD.

175. Wise men have declared, whosoever refrains from eating or drinking immoderately, and will only partake temperately perately of food and drink, as his constitution requires, shall enjoy health and long days, that is, a long life. Philosophers never said anything to the contrary. Desire, love, and the reception of worldly honour, these things fortify and assist life, so that they be gratified temperately. On which account, whosoever desireth life and permanence, let him seek that which is permanent and tends to prolong life.

MODERATION A MEANS TO PROLONG LIFE.—HIPPOCRATES AND HIS DISCIPLES.

176. Whosoever would prolong life, should restrain his appetite, and not eat over abundantly. I have heard that Ipocras1 having attained to old age, whereby he had to suffer much from infirmity and the weight of years, was addressed by his disciples, thus:—"Thou great teacher of wisdom, didst thou eat and drink abundantly, wouldst thou have to endure all the weakness which thou dost?" Then Ipocras:—"My sons, (said he) I eat a proper portion seeing I live, I should not live if (with a view of prolonging mere human life,) I partook of food too frequently. Eating is not the one thing needful, when the prolonging of life is the object aimed at, for I have seen many die from too much eating."

EAT SLOWLY AND SPARINGLY.— MEN OF ARABIA.— TWO RULES TO PRESERVE HEALTH.

177. Whosoever, restraining their appetite, refrain from gluttony, and eat slowly, these shall live long ; which may be thus proved. The men of Arabia, who dwell in mountains and pathless woods, are the most long lived (of mortals,) as these circumstances prevent excessive eating and drinking. The health may be preserved in two ways. First, — that is, by partaking of such food as is most suitable to the time of life and the constitution, restricting himself to that sort of diet which he was reared upon. Secondly, — by evacuating duly, what is poured into the stomach from above.

A THEORY OF DIGESTION.

178. Let all men know, that the human organism is antagonistic to food and drink, (decomposing both in the process of digestion,) and that every (animal or human) being is (naturally) verging upon disease. Also, animal organisms are corrupt from superabundant heat, which dries the spirit (anima) by which the body is nourished. Animal bodies also are corrupt from excessive heat of the sun, which dries the (animal) spirits ; and this is particularly the case with the bodies of the animals upon which we feed. When the body is hot, strong aliments are required, as then they can be digested.

FAT AND DRY CONSTITUTIONS.

179. When a (man's) body is fat and dry, luxurious juicy food is proper for him, for they will easily assimilate. 1n this way a man may preserve his health. Let him confine himself to such food as is suitable to his constitution. This has been proved.

A HOT HABIT.

180. If a man's body be constitutionally hot, hot aliment is proper for him.

A COLD HABIT.

181. If a man's body be constitutionally cold, cold aliments are proper for him.

A HUMID OR DRY HABIT.

182. If the body be constitutionally humid or.dry, cold aliments are forbidden him.

WHAT FOOD MOST SUITABLE FOR WEAK OR STRONG STOMACH.

183. Strong food is most suitable for a hot stomach, as such a stomach is comparable to fire consuming loose flax. Weak food is most proper for a cold stomach, as such a stomach is comparable to fire consuming straw.

HEALTHY DIGESTION.

184. The signs of a healthy digestion are, that the body be active, the understanding clear, and the desire for food frequent.

SYMPTOMS OF INDIGESTION.

185. The signs of indigestion are, heaviness of body, with irritability of feeling superadded, a languid performance of duty, swelling of the face, frequent yawning, dimness of sight, frequent eructations, attended with a bitterness of taste, (in the mouth,) this bitterness occasioning cardialgía, which extending to the body and limbs, occasions a dislike for food.

HOW TO ACT AT GETTING FROM BED, AND SUBSEQUENTLY DURING THE DAY, WITH OTHER HYGENIC MATTERS.

186. When rising from bed, walk a while, stretch your limbs, contracting your head and neck. This will strengthen your limbs, and the contracting of the head wlll cause the (animal) spirits to rush from the stomach to the head, and from the head, when you sleep, it will fall to the stomach again. In the summer, bathe in cold water, for this will keep warmth in the head, which will occasion a desire for food. Then array yourself in fair garments, for a man's mind delights in fair things, and his heart is rendered lighter. Then clean the teeth with the dry bark of the hazel, as they will become all the fairer in consequence. Your speech will be also most distinct, and breath sweeter. The standing posture should be at times practised, as it will do you much good, relieving the dura matter (membrane of the brain,) clothing your neck with power, investing your countenance with greater beauty, giving strength to the arms, improving your sight, preserving you from paleness, and adding power to your memory. Conversation, walking in company, and eating and drinking according to your usual habit, should be done in moderation. Use moderate exercise in walking or riding, as this will invigorate the body, and remove cardialgic pains, so that a man will be more hearty, strong, and the stomach will be. warmer as, well as your nerves more elastic.

WHAT TO EAT.

187. When you eat, take that for which you have the greatest relish if you can, particularly leavened bread. If you eat simple food it will be more easy for the stomach to digest it. If (when unused thereto) you should nevertheless eat two kinds of food, plain and strong food, eat the strong first, for the inferior portion of the stomach is hotter than the superior, as the lime is nearer, from whence more heat will be derived.

RULES FOR EATING AND DRINKING.

188. When you eat, do not eat away all your appetite, but let some desire for food remain. Drink no water with your food, as it will cool your stomach, preventing its digesting the food, and quenching the warmth thereof. But when you drink water, drink it sparingly, choosing the coldest water you can get. When you have done eating, take a walk in some well sheltered level piece of ground. When you feel inclined to sleep, do not sleep too much. Rest on your right side, then turn on the left, and double yourself. If you should feel pain in your stomach (cardialgía) and heaviness, put on extra clothing, in order to withdraw the heat from the stomach, drinking warm water, as this by producing vomiting will remove the unhealthy matter from your stomach. Walking much before food will heat the stomach. Much walking after food will injure the stomach, because undigested (in consequence of the labour) the food will fall to the inferior part of the stomach, and there generate many diseases. Sleeping before food will make a man thin, but sleeping after food will make a man fat. The night is colder than the day, and consequently the stomach will digest sooner by night than by day, because the colder the weather, the better will the stomach digest, as the heat falla from the extremities, and concentrates itself about the stomach. If a man who is in the habit of eating twice a day, should do so once only, it will injure the stomach. If a man in the habit of eating once only daily, should do so twice, it will be hurtful to the stomach. If from eating at one period of the day, we change to another, it will do harm to the stomach. At all times, if necessity should arise, obliging one to make a change in ones habit, let it be done gradually. Also do not eat, till the stomach has become empty, and this you may know from the sense of hunger and the thinness of your saliva. If you eat without hunger, the animal heat will freeze. If you eat when hungry, your

animal spirits will be as hot as fire, and whosoever does not then take food, his stomach will fill up with insalubrity, which will produce headache.

CPSIA information can be obtained
at www.ICGtesting.com
Printed in the USA
BVHW030327020822
643544BV00021B/2137